ALLERGIES

EXPLORING THE WORLD OF ALLERGIES

DR. J. SIMON

Table of Contents

INTRODUCTION 3

CHAPTER ONE 5

What Allergies Are 5

Categories of Allergies 7

Dietary allergies 8

Why and What's at Risk 12

The signs and symptoms.....................................17

CHAPTER TWO 20

A respiratory distress 20

Constitutional Signs and Symptoms..................21

Medical Evaluation and Diagnosis.....................22

Therapy Techniques 28

Here are some common approaches to allergy treatment:......28

A shift in lifestyle and education......................32

Things to Consider About Your Lifestyle 33

Recognize triggers and avoid them:.................34

An all-encompassing diet 37

CHAPTER THREE 40

Preparedness for Emergencies and Epidemics 40

CONCLUSION...45

THE END 49

INTRODUCTION

Allergies are a common, and frequently misinterpreted, immune system reaction to substances known as allergens. Some people have an overly strong immune response to these substances, but many others can tolerate them without any problems. There are many symptoms that can result from this hypersensitivity, ranging from minor irritation to severe, potentially fatal reactions.

Pollen, some foods, insect venom, animal dander, medications, and more can all contain allergens. Allergy sufferers experience symptoms like sneezing, itching, swelling, and in extreme situations, anaphylaxis, when their particular allergen is encountered by the immune system, which responds by releasing chemicals called histamines.

It's critical for people dealing with allergic reactions to comprehend allergies, their triggers, and practical management techniques. For efficient management and an enhanced quality of life, every type of allergy from food allergies to seasonal allergies requires specific insights and strategies.

CHAPTER ONE

What Allergies Are

As an elevated and aberrant immune reaction to substances that are generally safe for most people, allergies are caused by certain substances. For people who are sensitive to them or who are allergic, these substances, also referred to as allergens, can cause an allergic reaction. A variety of symptoms can arise from an allergic person's immune system misinterpreting certain substances as dangerous and reacting defensively.

Allergens that are frequently encountered in the home include dust mites, pollen, pet dander, insect stings, and specific foods (like dairy, nuts, and shellfish). Histamines are among the chemicals released by the immune system in allergic individuals in response to inhaling or coming into contact with these allergens. This is done to protect the body from foreign substances.

A person's immune system and the type of allergen they are exposed to can both influence how they react to allergens. Melting, itching, hives, swelling, nasal congestion, breathing difficulties, and, in severe cases, anaphylaxis—a potentially fatal reaction—are among the symptoms that can vary in severity.

Allergies can manifest at any age, and some people may eventually outgrow specific allergies. Individuals with known allergies frequently collaborate with healthcare professionals to identify triggers, prevent exposure, and effectively address symptoms because allergies are a chronic condition that requires ongoing management.

Categories of Allergies

A wide variety of allergens can cause allergies, which can manifest in different ways and impact different bodily systems. Some typical allergy types are as follows:

Allergies of the respiratory system:

Allergy-related symptoms such as sneezing, nasal congestion, itching, and watery eyes are caused by airborne allergens like mold spores, pollen, and pet dander. This condition is also known as hay fever (allergic rhinorrhea).

Asthma symptoms: Wheezing, shortness of breath, and tightness in the chest can be brought on by specific allergens such as mold, pollen, dust mites, or animal dander.

Dietary allergies

Anaphylactic shock is a severe allergic reaction that can result from a reaction to any number of foods, including wheat, eggs, milk, nuts, shellfish, and wheat.

Skin Intolerances:

Atopic dermatitis, also known as eczema, is characterized by red, itchy, and inflamed skin.

Eczema can be exacerbated by allergies to certain foods, fabrics, or dermatological products.

Contact dermatitis: Skin irritation can result from allergic reactions to materials such as certain metals, plants (like poison ivy), or chemicals in makeup.

An allergy to insect stings:

Insect stings, like those from bees, wasps, or ants, can cause life-threatening allergies in certain people. Localized swelling and anaphylaxis are examples of symptoms.

Hypersensitivity reactions to drugs:

Allergy-related reactions to drugs, like antibiotics, NSAIDs, or some anesthesia, can result in a variety of symptoms, like itching, skin rashes, or more severe reactions.

Allergies to latex:

Latex allergies can result in more serious symptoms such as skin irritation and hives when it comes to rubber products like gloves and balloons.

Allergies of the Eye:

Known as allergic conjunctivitis, allergic reactions that affect the eyes can result from exposure to allergens such as pollen or pet dander and cause redness, itching, and watering.

Allergies at Work:

Allergies resulting from occupational exposure to dust, fumes, or specific chemicals can strike certain people.

Hypersensitivity reactions to drugs:

Allergy-related reactions to drugs, like antibiotics, NSAIDs, or some anesthesia, can result in a variety of symptoms, like itching, skin rashes, or more severe reactions.

Physical Activity-Related Allergies:

A condition known as exercise-induced anaphylaxis occurs when a person exercises and experiences allergy-like symptoms, such as hives or difficulty breathing.

People should get tested and evaluated by doctors to determine which specific allergies they have. Understanding this helps prevent triggers, treat allergic reactions quickly when they happen, and manage allergies effectively.

Why and What's at Risk

An individual's lifestyle, environment, and genetic makeup can all play a role in how allergies develop. The risk of experiencing allergic reactions is increased by a number of factors, although the precise cause of allergies is not entirely known. These are typical causes of allergies as well as risk factors:

DNA Propensity:

The chance of someone acquiring allergies is higher in families where allergies run in the family. A person's susceptibility to allergic conditions can be influenced by genetic factors.

Antibodies of the Immune System:

The development of allergies is more common in people whose immune systems are hypersensitive or overactive. Toxic substances can cause the immune system to overreact and mistake them for threats.

Early Childhood Exposure:

Allergies may develop differently in children or infants who are exposed to allergens early on. One other factor associated with an increased risk is the absence of early exposure to specific substances, like peanuts or environmental allergens.

Elements of the Environment:

The development of allergies may be facilitated by exposure to environmental allergens such as dust mites, pollen, mold spores, pet dander, and insect venom.

Hygiene Theory:

According to the hygiene hypothesis, early childhood allergies may be more common in children who have had less exposure to germs and infectious agents. A child's immune system may be impacted by excessively sterile surroundings during childhood.

Factors relating to lifestyle:

Some aspects of living, like residing in cities, not doing a lot of outdoor activities, and being more exposed to indoor pollutants, can affect the development of allergies.

Nutritional Considerations:

The development of food allergies can be influenced by early dietary decisions, such as breastfeeding and the introduction of solid foods. A higher risk might result from introducing some foods later than others.

Occupational Hazards:

The development of occupational allergies may be facilitated by exposure to allergens or irritants in certain types of work.

Place of Geographical Location:

Regional variations in environmental factors and allergy prevalence are possible. People with hay fever, for instance, might be more likely to live in areas with high pollen counts.

cigarette use and air pollution:

There is evidence linking the development of respiratory allergies to exposure to air pollution and tobacco smoke.

Past Sensitivity to allergens:

The likelihood of developing allergies to other substances is higher in people who have previously experienced allergic reactions.

Not everyone with these risk factors will experience allergic conditions, despite the fact that they increase the likelihood of allergies.

Each person's experience with allergies is unique and can be complicated. A medical evaluation and testing are essential for an accurate diagnosis and suitable management if a person suspects they have allergies or experiences allergic reactions.

The signs and symptoms

Various symptoms and bodily systems may be impacted by allergic reactions. Allergy symptoms can vary in intensity, with the type of allergen and the person's immune system determining the exact symptoms. The following list includes typical allergy symptoms:

Symptoms of the respiratory system:

Sneezing: When exposed to airborne allergens such as pollen or pet dander, frequent and sudden sneezing is a common symptom.

Swollen or Runny Nose: Respiratory allergies can cause postnasal drip, runny nose, and nasal congestion.

Dry or Watery Eyes: Common symptoms of airborne allergens include dryness, redness, irritation, and excessive tearing.

Signs and symptoms of the skin:

Hives (Urticaria): Food allergies, insect stings, or medication-induced skin irritations can cause elevated, itchy welts to develop.

The skin condition known as eczema (atopic dermatitis) is characterized by red, itchy, and inflamed skin. Allergies can cause eczema to develop or worsen.

Illnesses of the Stomach:

stomach ache: Food allergies or intolerances can cause stomach ache or discomfort in certain people.

nauseous vomiting: Nausea and vomiting can be caused by allergic reactions to specific foods or drugs.

CHAPTER TWO

A respiratory distress

Coughing: Respiratory allergens or irritants may cause people to cough persistently.

Wheezing is a common respiratory symptom of asthma that is brought on by allergens. It is caused by constriction of the airways.

An allergy reaction:

Swelling: More serious allergic reactions can result in sudden, severe swelling, particularly of the lips, tongue, and face.

Breathlessness: Breathing problems, dyspnea, and a constricted chest are all possible outcomes of anaphylaxis.

Dizziness or unconsciousness may result from a sharp drop in blood pressure brought on by severe allergic reactions.

Constitutional Signs and Symptoms

Fatigue: Exhaustion can be a result of allergic reactions, particularly when there is inflammation present.

Malaise: Allergy reactions can be accompanied by a generalized discomfort or unease.

Noting that allergy reactions can range widely in severity and that anaphylaxis can occasionally be fatal and necessitate immediate medical attention are important points to remember. Medical attention should be sought immediately if a person exhibits severe symptoms, such as breathing difficulties or facial swelling. People who have established allergies should work with medical professionals to develop a customized management plan. This plan may involve avoidance methods and drugs like antihistamines or adrenaline for severe reactions.

Medical Evaluation and Diagnosis

The standard methods for diagnosing allergies are a physical examination, a medical history, and sometimes allergy testing. The steps involved in diagnosing and evaluating allergies medically are summarized as follows:

Background information on health:

In order to determine the kind and pattern of symptoms, medical professionals need to obtain a complete medical history. Concerns regarding the types of symptoms experienced, their duration, and any potential patterns or triggers will be discussed with them.

Evaluation of the body:

A physical examination may be done to find out how the patient is feeling generally and to look for any obvious signs of an allergic reaction, such as skin rashes or breathing difficulties.

Performing an allergy test:

A tiny amount of allergen extracts is applied to the skin using a tiny needle in the well-known allergy test known as the "Skin Prick Test." Someone who is allergic to a particular medication at the test site may get a little raised bump, or hive.

Testing for specific antibodies (IgE) that the body produces in response to allergens can be done using serum IgE, or blood, tests. Common blood tests for allergies screening include the RAST and ImmunoCAP tests.

Patch tests are carried out to identify the allergens that cause contact dermatitis. After applying and leaving the patches on the skin for a pre-arranged period of time, patches containing minute amounts of potential allergens are applied.

Diet of Elimination:

A suspected food allergy may require the use of an elimination diet. This involves taking particular foods out of the diet and gradually reintroducing them in order to find possible triggers.

Trials of Difficulty:

A supervised, medically monitored exposure to potential allergens is required for challenge testing. To confirm or rule out specific dietary sensitivities, these tests are commonly carried out.

Tongue endoscopy:

When there are respiratory allergies, a nasal endoscopy can be performed to look for signs of inflammation or allergic rhinitis in the nasal passages.

Examinations for Lung Health:

Spirometry and other lung function tests may be used to assess airway function in patients suspected of having respiratory allergies or asthma.

Diagnostic imaging:

Diagnostic imaging methods such as CT scans and chest X-rays can be used in some situations to evaluate how allergens affect the respiratory system.

Record of Symptoms and Medical Background:

A symptom diary, wherein the onset and nature of symptoms are noted, could be requested of the public. With the use of this data, identifying patterns and triggers will be simpler.

Symptoms and potential triggers must be discussed openly and honestly with medical professionals. When an accurate diagnosis is obtained, a personalized treatment plan can be created that includes lifestyle modifications, medication (such as antihistamines or epinephrine), and allergy avoidance. Treating allergy diseases may be more specifically explained by speaking with an immunologist or allergist.

Reducing allergen exposure, symptomatically, and, in some cases, modulating the immune system are the objectives of treating allergies. Treatment options may vary depending on the type and severity of allergies.

Here are some common approaches to allergy treatment:

Keeping Allergens at Bay:

Identifying and staying away from allergens is a crucial component of allergy management. Making lifestyle adjustments to stay away from recognized triggers, using air purifiers, and maintaining a hypoallergenic home are some ways to achieve this.

Drugs:

Antihistamines: By blocking histamine's effects, these medications help lessen symptoms like runny nose, sneezing, and itching.

Decongestants: These medications may provide brief relief from nasal congestion by narrowing blood vessels and reducing edema.

Nasal Steroids: Due to their ability to decrease nasal canal irritation, corticosteroid nasal sprays are effective in treating allergic rhinitis.

Inhaled bronchodilators may be recommended for individuals experiencing allergic-triggered asthma episodes.

For severe allergic reactions, such as anaphylaxis, an epinephrine auto-injector may be used. Utilizing this intervention in an emergency situation could potentially save lives.

Vaccination (allergy shots or sublingual tablets):

A patient receiving small, controlled doses of allergens is used in immunotherapy to gradually desensitize their immune system. This can be administered sublingually, or under the tongue, with allergy injections.

ORT, or oral immunotherapy:

If you have particular food sensitivities, you might want to think about oral immunotherapy. This involves introducing the allergen gradually in small, controlled doses in order to build tolerance.

Combinations of Medication for Allergies:

To treat multiple allergy symptoms at once, some medications combine decongestants and antihistamines.

Topical Interventions:

Topical Steroids: To relieve inflammation caused by skin allergies or eczema, topical corticosteroid creams or ointments can be applied topically.

Topically applied topical antihistamines can help lessen the itching and discomfort associated with skin allergies.

Drops of the eye:

When allergic conjunctivitis occurs, antihistamine eye drops can help lessen the redness, irritation, and itching.

A shift in lifestyle and education

People can recognize their triggers and modify their lifestyles to minimize their exposure by learning more about allergies. It might mean changing one's diet, keeping an eye on pollen counts, and avoiding certain places.

Emergency Protocol:

Serious allergy sufferers should have an emergency plan in place, especially if they are prone to anaphylaxis. An auto-injector of epinephrine may be used in accordance with this strategy, which outlines what to do in case of a severe allergic reaction.

Individuals with allergies, in particular immunologists and allergists, should work closely with healthcare professionals to develop a personalized treatment plan. Periodic follow-ups and plan adjustments may be necessary, contingent on the patient's response to treatment and the variability of their allergen exposure.

Things to Consider About Your Lifestyle

A few targeted lifestyle modifications can help manage allergies and lessen the frequency and severity of allergic responses. For individuals with allergies, consider these lifestyle recommendations:

Find out which specific allergens are causing your symptoms by working with medical professionals. Make a conscious effort to avoid these triggers once you've identified them.

Create an Environment That Is Hypoallergenic at Home:

Use techniques such as air purifiers, hot water laundry, and window coverings during high pollen seasons to reduce allergens in your home.

Resolve indoor air quality issues:

Fit HVAC systems and air purifiers with high-efficiency particulate air (HEPA) filters to capture allergens in the air. Dusting and cleaning your home frequently will help to reduce indoor allergens.

Monitor your pollen concentrations:

Especially during peak season, stay informed about local pollen counts. Try to limit your time outside and wear sunglasses to protect your eyes on days when pollen counts are high.

Construct an Allergy-Proof Bedroom:

Pick mattresses and pillowcases that are allergen-proof to reduce your exposure to dust mites. Do hot water routine laundry for bedding, drapes, and carpets.

Supplies for Personal Hygiene:

Choose hypoallergenic and fragrance-free personal care products to lessen skin sensitivity. Make sure you carefully read the labels of makeup, lotions, and soaps to avoid potential allergies.

Avoid smoking and being around smoke:

When someone smokes or is around someone who smokes, asthma and respiratory allergies can exacerbate. Stay away from smoke-filled areas and avoid smoking yourself.

Sustain Your Hydration:

Eating a healthy diet rich in water also helps prevent dehydration and relieve the pain associated with irritated or dry mucal membranes.

To support your immune system's overall health, keep a nutritious, well-balanced diet. When it comes to people who have specific food allergies, dietary adjustments may be recommended.

Frequent Exercise:

Engage in moderate exercise on a regular basis to improve your overall health and cardiovascular health. Before starting a new fitness program, consult with medical professionals.

Regulate Your Tension:

When under stress, allergy symptoms may worsen. Take up stress-relieving exercises like yoga, meditation, or deep breathing to help lower your stress levels.

Acquire Personal Knowledge:

Stay up to date on allergies, triggers, and treatments that are available. Being health-conscious enables you to prevent and control allergic reactions before they happen.

Emergency Protocol:

Anyone with severe allergies should have an emergency plan, especially if they are at risk of suffering anaphylaxis. Guidelines on how to use an auto-injector of epinephrine in case of a severe allergic reaction should be included in this plan.

Remember that you can develop a personalized lifestyle plan that addresses your specific allergy symptoms and triggers by consulting with medical professionals, especially immunologists or allergists. As allergen exposure and patient reactions change, routine checkups can help modify the treatment plan.

CHAPTER THREE

Preparedness for Emergencies and Epidemics

It's crucial to be ready for anything unexpected when dealing with severe allergies, particularly for those who may experience anaphylaxis, a severe and occasionally fatal allergic reaction. Treating anaphylaxis promptly is necessary because it can occur suddenly. When managing anaphylaxis and getting ready for emergencies, remember the following:

Auto-Injector of Epinephrine:

It is advisable for people who have previously suffered from severe allergies, especially to foods, insect stings, or medications, to always carry an auto-injector of epinephrine. With this device, anaphylactic symptoms can be promptly treated with the potentially lethal medication epinephrine.

Proficiency in Using the Auto-Injector:

Make certain that the allergy sufferer and anyone close to them, such as friends, family, or caregivers, are proficient in using the epinephrine auto-injector. Training may be provided by healthcare professionals.

More than one injector for the auto:

Ensure you have extra auto-injectors available in case you need to give higher doses of epinephrine for severe allergic reactions. When an electronic device reaches its expiration date, replace it immediately.

Establish an emergency action plan:

Along with medical professionals, create a personalized emergency action plan that outlines what to do in the event of an allergic reaction. Share this tactic with the staff at the school, your friends, family, and coworkers.

Put a medical ID on:

Make sure everyone knows what allergies you have and how likely you are to experience anaphylaxis by wearing a medical alert necklace or bracelet. This information may be vital for emergency responders.

Notify Nearby Partners:

Those who have frequent contact with the person should be made aware of their allergies and know what to do in an emergency, such as friends, family, and coworkers.

Assess Symptoms of Anaphylaxis:

Be aware of the warning signs and symptoms of anaphylaxis, which include throat or face swelling, hives, gastrointestinal issues, a drop in blood pressure, and trouble breathing. If any of these indicators show up, act right away.

Put in a call for emergency assistance:

In case of a severe allergic reaction, immediately contact emergency services. We need to get medical help right away because time is of the essence.

Hold yourself together and lie down:

Remain calm and lay down if you suspect you are experiencing anaphylaxis. Circumstances that cause stress may exacerbate symptoms. To improve blood circulation, try elevating your legs.

Give yourself an adrenaline auto-injector if you are able to and instructed to do so while you wait for emergency help. As soon as possible, administer it; delaying its use could have negative consequences.

Continually Provide Emergency Medical Attention:

Receive emergency medical attention as soon as possible, even if administering epinephrine relieves symptoms. Careful assessment and ongoing observation are required in cases of anaphylaxis.

Anaphylaxis control requires prompt action and the possession of an emergency plan. Patients with severe allergies need to be well-prepared for emergencies by keeping track of new developments in allergy management therapies, communicating with medical professionals on a regular basis, and updating their emergency action plan frequently.

CONCLUSION

In summary, allergies are intricate immunological reactions to mostly benign chemicals referred to as allergens. They can affect the gastrointestinal tract, skin, respiratory system, and other organs in diverse ways. Allergies affect people of all ages, ranging from moderate hay fever to severe food allergies, and they necessitate careful management and lifestyle adjustments.

A comprehensive assessment that includes a physical examination, medical history, and, in certain situations, allergy testing is required to diagnose allergies. Effective treatment plans are based on the particular type and degree of allergies and are customized after diagnosis. These could include avoiding allergens, using drugs like epinephrine or antihistamines, immunotherapy, and changing one's way of living.

The way one lives affects how one manages their allergies. The three main ways to improve general health are by recognizing and avoiding triggers, making hypoallergenic settings, and keeping track of pollen counts. Emergency readiness includes developing an emergency action plan, teaching close contacts, and carrying and operating an epinephrine auto-injector, especially for those who are at risk of anaphylaxis.

Although managing allergies needs constant attention to detail, new developments in allergy research and therapy continue to raise hopes for better quality of life and better management. People with allergies can minimize the impact of allergic responses on their daily activities and lead satisfying and healthy lives by collaborating closely with healthcare experts, remaining informed, and taking proactive measures.

THE END